6 Healing Movements

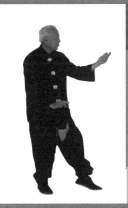

6 HEALING MOVEMENTS

Qigong

FOR
HEALTH
STRENGTH
LONGEVITY

Master Gin Foon Mark

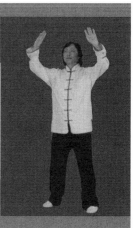

YMAA PUBLICATION CENTER
Boston, Mass. USA

YMAA PUBLICATION CENTER
Main Office: 4354 Washington Street
Boston, Massachusetts, 02131
617-323-7215; ymaa@aol.com
www.ymaa.com

Printed in Canada
10 9 8 7 6 5 4 3 2 1

Cover design by Katya Popova

ISBN: 1-886969-90-6

Publisher's Cataloging in Publication

(Prepared by Quality Books Inc.)

Mark, Gin Foon.
  Six healing movements of qigong : for health,
strength, longevity / Gin Foon Mark. — 1st ed.
  p. cm.
  Includes index.
  ISBN: 1-886969-90-6

  1. Qi gong—Therapeutioc use. I. Title.

RA781.8.M37 2001   615.8'2
                         QBI01-201021

Disclaimer:

The authors and publisher of this material are not responsible in any manner whatsoever for any injury which may occur through reading or following the instructions in this manual. The activities, physical or otherwise, described in this material may be too strenuous or dangerous for some people, and the reader(s) should consult a physician before engaging in them.

I would like to give my deepest thank you to my daughters Paula and Roxy, and to my devoted wife Juanita, for their help in making this book possible.

養生氣功
六字訣、

Contents

Foreword

I am honored to have the opportunity to comment on two genuine treasures in my life: Six Healing Sounds Qigong and Master Gin Foon Mark. I first began my studies with Master Mark in 1986, and have been privileged to train with him in Qigong, Gongfu, and Chinese brush painting, as well as enjoying the full range of his marvelous cooking skills. I have found in him that paradoxical combination of indisputable mastery and self-confidence in his own skills contrasted with genuine humility, a joy and openness in sharing his knowledge, and a heartwarming sense of humor.

Master Mark's lineage and accomplishments are too extensive to list here except in briefest outline. Born into a family with a rich martial arts heritage in pre-communist China, he studied the full range of martial, medical, meditation, cooking, and fine arts with renowned martial artists in his own family and in several temples in China and Macao. He continued as teacher and student after his move to New York in 1947 where he concentrated on, and was eventually designated Master of, the Southern Praying Mantis Gongfu system. Master Mark learned Six Healing Sounds Qigong from its originator, "Old Man" Ma Laitong, on his subsequent travels back to Beijing.

Qigong is one of the more recently popularized Chinese mind/body arts. It joins the arts of Gongfu, Chinese Medicine/Acupuncture, Taiji, Feng Shui, etc. in commanding the interest and fascination of many Americans eager for activities and perspectives that go beyond the traditional Western paradigms. As is typical of our culture, when a subject gains mass interest, the market is deluged with books, videos, and classes from myriad teachers looking to satisfy that new interest. While the majority of these new teachers undoubtedly offer valuable information to the public, it is exceedingly rare to have the opportunity to learn from a true master of the art.

I have found Six Healing Sounds Qigong to be one of the most beneficial and easily learned forms of the art. Besides notable enhancement of my energy level and general well-being, practice of this Qigong brought about the resolution of a nagging physical condition that had not previously responded to yoga, taiji, or massage therapy. I also believe that routine practice can have a significant balancing effect on female hormone levels. This has potential effects on PMS, menopause, and even fertility.

Master Mark's students all have stories of "Qigong" babies, conceived after the mothers or couples began Qigong training. While having a new baby may not be the goal of most readers of this book, I do wish everyone the birthing of new possibilities for physical and mental health through the practice of Six Healing Sounds Qigong.

Dr. James J. Rosamilia, Jr.
Minnesota, November 2000

About the Author

Gin Foon Mark was born in 1927 in Toison, China, a small village near Canton (Guandong). At the age of five he began his studies in the art of Gongfu, under the supervision of his uncle Kong Boon Fu, a 4th generation master of White Crane Gongfu. His grandfather, who was also a master, tutored him in their family style known as Mok Gar (Mark Style) Gongfu.

At the age of nine he was admitted to the Shaolin Temple at Chun San and studied with the monk Moot Ki Fut Sai. During his stay in the Shaolin Temple Master Mark received instruction in the Five Animal Style, White Crane, Eagle Claw, Leopard, and Tiger Gongfu styles.

While in the Shaolin Temple he learned many external and internal Qigong exercises, including Iron Shirt, Iron Palm and Cotton Palm. He also learned acupuncture techniques for healing.

In 1947 the Chinese Association of New York asked Master Mark to come to the United States to teach Gongfu to the Chinese community. In 1956, at the age of 29, Gin Foon Mark began studying under Lum Wing Fai, the fourth generation master of the Southern Praying Mantis Gongfu system. For the next 13 years he studied with Master Lum. In 1969 Master Lum closed his hands (retired) and appointed Master Mark to take over as the fifth generation master of this system.

Master Mark opened Southern Praying Mantis Gongfu schools in New York and Philadelphia. In 1970 he moved to Minnesota and also opened a school in Minneapolis. Master Mark is now living in St. Paul, Minnesota and teaching daily classes.

In 1979 Master Mark went back to China. While he was there he studied Six Healing Sounds Qigong in Beijing under a teacher known as the "Old Master of China". Master Mark gained much valuable knowledge from his study of many Qigong styles, so he decided to share his knowledge and experience by teaching the "Six Healing Sounds" to students in his Gongfu school.

Master Mark is also an accomplished Chinese ink-brush artist and calligrapher. He has been featured on the national television program "You Asked for It." The State of Minnesota holds Master Mark in high esteem and has produced a videotape of him that is included in the collection of their State Cultural Treasure Program.

Master Mark is now writing a book on the Southern Praying Mantis Gongfu system.

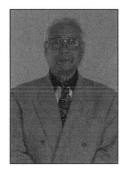

Gin Foon Mark, Author

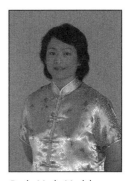

Paula Mark, Model

How to Use this Book

This book was designed to give you an introduction to the art of Qigong and a step-by-step guide to follow when doing the Qigong exercises.

First read through the book and familiarize yourself with the concepts. Then re-read the book, underlining the important passages that interest you. When you feel you understand the concepts and are familiar with how to do the exercises, you may begin the exercises, keeping the book near at hand. Check the book often, especially when you are not sure that you are doing the exercises correctly.

Read this book carefully and follow the exercises exactly. Do not take shortcuts in your practice. If at all possible, take lessons from a qualified instructor who will demon- strate, instruct, and make suggestions and corrections when necessary. Some of the ideas inherent to Qigong are best taught and explained by an instructor. Books are better used for background information and to supplement the instruction of a qualified teacher.

Qigong is an art you will use for the rest of your life. As you begin to learn the concepts, avoid becoming impatient while awaiting results. Sometimes beginners expect results overnight. Qigong takes time, practice, and patience. As time passes you will see the benefits of your Qigong practice. Success depends solely on you, and on your perseverance in doing the exercises daily. If you take the time to practice the Six Healing Sounds Qigong daily, you can experience results in as little as two weeks.

Keep an open mind as you read this book and above all else have fun and enjoy yourself.

Editor's Note

Since its inception several thousand years ago, Qigong has been passed down from Master to Sifu to student, from man to man to man. Traditionally the masters and practitioners of the Chinese healing and martial arts were men. But during the twentieth century, when these arts were allowed to leave China, they became available to members of both sexes, in China and the world over, and more women began to practice and eventually teach. Note that the practitioner shown in the photos is a woman. YMAA assigned us to work together as a team so that we could strike the balance required to present the subject as universally as possible, balancing the yin and yang (female and male) considerations as best we can.

As a woman practicing Qigong for the last fifteen years, I can attest to the fact that these practices can be as beneficial to women as they are to men. I must point out however that there are still many principles directed at the male anatomy and condition that are just now being addressed from the female perspective. In the section in Chapter 3 entitled "When Not to Practice" Master Mark's instructions regarding practice during menstruation are specific, but other female issues are being studied as they arise, and some have even yet to be considered. My advice to all women is to pay close attention to your bodies' responses to these, or any, exercises. In the case of pregnant women, you must consult your doctors before beginning Qigong, just as you would before undertaking any new exercise system.

YMAA provides us with the tools to learn and improve. In everything that we do, each of us, male and female alike, bears the ultimate responsibility for listening to his or her own body and proceeding appropriately.

Lynn Teale
Editor

CHAPTER 1
INTRODUCTION

What is Qigong?

Qigong is a system for curing and preventing illness and stress, and for enhancing all aspects of life. Its key concept is that of increasing our vital energy, or Qi, through easy techniques and physical exercise. This life force energy is circulated through the acupuncture meridians of the body. Qi is the continuous flow of energy that links the various tissues, organs, and brain functions that result in a whole, unified person.

Qigong, also properly called Nei Gong (internal Gongfu), means the skills for training and maneuvering the breath by the mind.

Qi, in Chinese medicine, is everything from the air we breathe to the vital energy that animates our bodies. Kung, or Gong, means hard work, patience, and dedication over a long period of time. So, Qigong means the development of the body's energy circulation to both increase and control it.

Breath is the source of life. When we stop breathing, the body dies and becomes just an inanimate corpse. Since the nervous system no longer works, the mind vanishes and life comes to an end. Thus we know that a human being is made physically of a body and a mind, and that breath gives life to this being, playing an important role in uniting the two components.

This Qi is the primordial life force itself. It begins in human life with the piercing of an egg by a sperm cell. From this original fusion an enormously complex new human being develops. The fetus grows around its mother's navel point, and through its own navel absorbs nutrients and expels waste. The fetus literally breathes through the umbilical cord (prenatal Qi) from the mother into its own navel. The navel point is thus said by Daoists to be the starting point for the flow of this primordial life energy, or Qi, and remains the point of strongest energy storage and circulation of qi. Postnatal Qi can be classified into two kinds, heavenly Qi, the Qi (air) we inhale and exhale, and earthly Qi, the food we eat from the earth. Only when filled with both heavenly and earthly Qi can the human body carry on its vital activities.

Qi is one of the three principles upon which life depends. Qi is the force, or energy, of life. Jing is the heart of life, and

Shen is the light. Jing, Qi, and Shen are separate in human life but they can merge into one another. Jing functions in the lower abdomen, the kidneys, and genital organs. Qi functions in the chest, and Shen functions in the brain. The feelings of an orgasm come from Jing, determination, power, and firmness come from Qi, and wisdom comes from Shen.

Another concept involved in Qigong is the concept of Yin and Yang. In the beginning Yin and Yang originally meant darkness and lightness, but over time the Chinese have divided all things into Yin and Yang. Man and women, action and non-action, hard and soft, inner and outer, and up and down to name just a few. There is nothing in the universe that is purely Yin or Yang, everything has a little of its opposite inherent in it. In the practice of Qigong one learns to harmonize the Yin and Yang. One strives to put the body in harmony with its own Yin and Yang. All the postures and exercises that are the basis of Qigong are directed towards the goal of achieving harmony within one's self. For thousands of years Chinese physicians have believed that a long and peaceful life depends on the harmony one achieves in one's life, the harmony between Yin and Yang, and the harmonious flow of the life's energy (Qi).

You have probably heard of Muslim fakirs, who eat live scorpions and writhing snakes, of Indian yogis who walk on red-hot stones, or of Tibetan hermits who sit naked amid the Himalayan snows, yet feel no sense of cold. You may have seen martial arts exhibitions where a person will lay on a bed of nails with a concrete block resting on his stomach, and then someone will hit the block with a sledge hammer, with no ill effects to the one laying on the nails. All of these people have achieved remarkable control over their bodies through hard and long practice of Qigong breathing exercises, the results of which have altered the frailty of the human body and raised its power of resistance to an astonishing degree.

HISTORY OF QIGONG

In Chinese history, the first mention of a system of movements used to maintain health and to cure diseases dates back to prehistoric times, during the reign of the Great Yu. Emperor Yu instituted the dances named "Da Wu" or the Great Dances.

The history of "Qi" theory starts with the beginning of Chinese medicine during the reign of the Yellow Emperor Huang Di (2697-2597 B.C.) when he wrote *The Yellow Emperor's Classic of Medicine*. The Yellow Emperor's system was based on the use of herbs, acupuncture, massage, and systems of movements.

In the sixth century B.C., the philosopher Lao Zi, in his classic the *Dao De Jing*, described breathing techniques for increasing the life span. This was the first record of the use of breathing techniques to increase Qi circulation that, as a result, increased the length and quality of life.

During the Han Dynasty (206 B.C.–A.D. 220), the medical doctor Hua Tuo developed a system of therapy that used the movements of the bear, the deer, the monkey, the tiger, and the bird.

During the Liang dynasty (A.D. 502–557), a Buddhist monk, named Da Mo arrived at the Shaolin Temple. Da Mo saw that the monks were weak, could not concentrate for long, and could do very little. He pondered the problem and later wrote the *Yi Jin Jing* (muscle development classic). In this book he stressed concentration to develop local Qi and increase Qi circulation. The monks practiced these methods and found that they greatly increased their power, their ability to meditate for longer periods of time, and the length of their lives. These exercises were then turned into a system of self-defense. This was the first known application of Qigong to the martial arts.

Until 50 years ago little was known of Qigong, because most Qigong masters would teach only their own sons, or a few close, trusted friends. Many of the Qigong exercises were developed by Buddhist and Daoist monks who did not spread their teachings beyond their own temples. Because most people were kept ignorant of Qigong, it has been superstitiously regarded as magic.

How Qigong Is Used for Healing

According to traditional Chinese medicine, illness is caused by the blockage, or stagnation, of energy. Too much or too little energy in one part of the body results in disease to that part and stresses the entire body. Chinese medicine believes that negative emotions such as anger, fear, or cruelty, and excessive amounts of positive emotions such as joy or excitement can injure the organs and cause disease. Qigong exercises can cure such imbalances by awakening the Qi, or vital energy, and circulating it to the needed areas. By learning how to increase the Qi, we will have more Qi to open the blockages, increase the body's defensive powers, and prevent illness.

One of the most universal effects of continued Qigong practice is improved digestive function. Improved digestion occurs because the movement of the diaphragm while breathing massages the visceral organs and stimulates the function of the stomach and intestines, thereby improving digestion and absorption.

In recent studies in China, Qigong therapy has been

proven effective for the treatment of a wide variety of diseases and conditions including anxiety, hypertension, ulcers, high blood pressure, and chronic constipation.

WHY STUDY QIGONG?

We spend all our energy and money making certain that our outer selves are presentable, but we abuse our inner selves by overeating, eating an imbalanced diet, drinking, smoking, or denying ourselves love. Then we're shocked when our lungs collapse, we suffer a heart attack, our kidneys fail, or we are told we have cancer. Some people have an astonishing ability to convince themselves that their health is not caused by their own behavior, and quickly blame their illness on bad genes, old age, fate, etc. But most people are simply unaware that their illnesses are the direct result of years of accumulated stress and that the seemingly minor abuse

of their physical bodies can damage their vital organs.

As we age, the energy routes that bring vital power to our internal organs and enable them to function become progressively more blocked by physical and mental tension. The result is general fatigue, weakness, and poor health. If we do not live healthfully and practice Qigong to keep the energy routes open, these energy routes will gradually close and cause emotional imbalances, premature sickness, and premature aging.

Simply by reestablishing the same strong flow of Qi that we had as children, our vital organs will begin to glow with radiant health. Our true task is only to reawaken this healing power.

Most of us own an automobile and use it everyday to get from here to there. Several times a year we take it to someone to have it tuned up, the oil changed, the tires, battery, and coolant checked. We do this in the hope that our car will start more easily, last longer, and cost us less in repair bills over the years ahead. But what do we do for our own bodies? Do we give them the best fuel possible in the way of foods? Do we keep them from getting dirty by not smoking? Do we "change the oil," getting rid of the old air by doing breathing exercises and meditation? Do we see a doctor at a prescribed interval for a checkup? The answer to most, if not all, of these questions is probably "No." The average person is actually likely to spend more time and money caring for his or her car than caring for his or her own body. This book is a step-by-step manual to help you take care of yourself as well as you take care of your car.

ABOUT SIX HEALING SOUNDS QIGONG

Thousands of years ago the Daoist masters discovered sounds that were the correct frequencies to keep the organs in optimal condition. Qi flow was observed to be closely related to these sounds. Using careful observation the six sounds that corresponded with the organs of the body were found. To accompany the Six Healing Sounds, six accompanying postures were developed to activate the acupuncture meridians and energy channels of the organs.

The Six Healing Sounds work by speeding up the heat exchange from the different organs, moving the heat through the digestive system and then allowing it to escape from the mouth. As the sound is being made, the heat given off by the organ is transferred up the esophagus to leave the body as the sound is emitted from the mouth.

THE TEACHER (SIFU)

In studying any art, particularly Qigong, it is important to have a competent instructor who will monitor your progress, explain and demonstrate the exercises, correct you when you are doing them improperly, and give you new concepts when he or she feels you are ready to advance.

The teacher is there to motivate the student, to see that the student follows a proven path in the study of the art. The teacher is there to see that the student practices as much as possible under his or her supervision.

The Chinese believe that you insult your teacher if you undervalue the lesson, by not practicing to the best of your ability. If you practice only a little and then want the teacher to show you something new, you are indicating to your Sifu that you do not appreciate his or her instruction. The novice student should spend as much time as possible under the guidance of his or her Sifu.

The following sensations are commonly experienced in Qigong practice:

- Different parts of the body may experience itching or tingling.

- Certain parts of the body may feel heavy.

- Heat or coolness may develop in different parts of the body.

- The body may feel as if it is floating, or possibly falling.

- Perspiration may appear on the hands and/or feet.

Remember:
There is no need to be concerned about these effects. Pay them as little attention as possible and they will soon vanish.

CHAPTER 2

GENERAL GUIDELINES OF QIGONG

BASIC GUIDELINES

No matter what deep breathing exercises you train in, you must master the art of regulating the mind, the breath, and the body.

Regulating the mind means that you allow your mind to relax into a state of tranquility, where you will, as much as possible, eliminate all thoughts that intrude as you do the exercises.

Regulating the breath means regulating the respiration and making it flow naturally, smoothly, slowly, and evenly.

Regulating the body means that all exercises are performed in the correct posture, requiring the entire body to be relaxed and natural.

The benefits you attain from Qigong primarily depend on your ability to become relaxed and tranquil. Whether the posture is correct, or whether the regulation of the breath is proper, will also directly affect the mind's ability to attain a relaxed state.

Regulating the mind, breath, and body will enable you to increase your vital energy and spirit, bringing your body's latent energy into play. This allows you to achieve the aim of strengthening the physique and enhancing your resistance against diseases.

In Summary: You must not force the motions but should let them happen naturally. At first the movements will feel awkward and unnatural, but through constant practice the body and mind will become

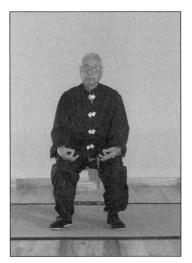

figure 2-1

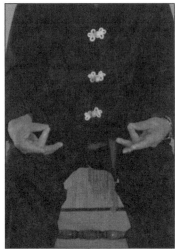

figure 2-2

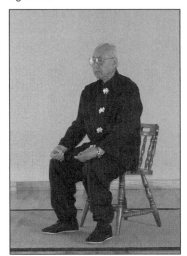

figure 2-3

accustomed to the movements, eventually allowing them to feel relaxed and natural. You must use as little force as possible while doing the exercises. To remain calm and relaxed with the mind concentrated is the key to Qigong. Do not talk with others while you train.

POSTURES

Although it is not necessary to practice all three of this chapter's Qigong postures during the same session, if you were to practice all three, the ideal sequence would begin with the sitting posture, followed by the standing posture, and finishing with the sleeping posture. But no matter what posture or postures you practice, the major criteria for your choice of posture should be your ability to remain completely relaxed, to be able to relax all your muscles, and to breathe in a relaxed and natural way. Most often the posture that feels the best for you is the best posture for you to practice.

When the posture is correct, Qi will flow freely.

If you feel any discomfort in any part of your body during practice, correct your posture or bring the exercise to a close.

sitting posture

The most important thing to remember is to keep the spinal cord straight and free of tension.

Sit up straight on the edge of the chair (figures 2-1 to 2-3). Do not incline to either side. Straighten the neck. Relax the waist, back, chest, and abdomen. Keep the head upright, as if it were suspended from above. The face should be slightly forward. Pull the chest in slightly and loosen the shoulders by dropping both elbows. Bend both knees. Place the feet shoulder width apart with both feet flat on the ground.

Remember:

It is important that the chair be the right height so that your knees are bent at a right angle and your thighs are parallel to the floor.

Do not lean back against the chair at any time.

Do not allow the lower back to curve backward in a slouch or forward to cause the abdomen to protrude.

standing posture

The standing posture (figure 2-4) is the main posture in Qigong.

Standing, when done properly, is an important form of exercise. In order to stand in a relaxed manner, one must use the force of gravity. The force of gravity acts downward. If the body, from the top of the head to the bottom of the feet, is visualized as if it were dangling from a string like a puppet, it will automatically follow the force of gravity.

Guidelines for the Standing Posture:

Head: Hold the head as if it were suspended by a rope from the heavens. Keep the head from tilting from side to side and front to back.

Eyes: Relax the eyes and let the upper lids droop naturally.

Tongue: The tongue should be touching the upper palate during inhalation and dropped down during exhalation.

Chin: Tuck in the chin.

Neck: Relax the neck (circle the head a few times to loosen the neck muscles).

Shoulders: Relax the shoulder joints and let them droop naturally.

Chest: Relax the chest. The chest should bend slightly forward thereby relaxing the diaphragm.

Elbows: Relax the elbows and hold them slightly away from the body in order to form hollows in the armpits.

Hands and fingertips: Are relaxed and at ease.

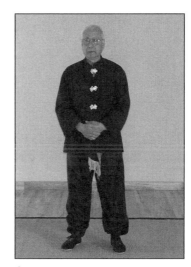

figure 2-4

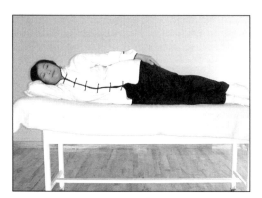

figure 2-5

Waist: Relax the waist and hips. When the waist is relaxed the spine will stand upright. To relax the waist lift up both shoulders, then relax them downward giving a big sigh (exhalation) as they drop down.

Stomach: Relax the entire abdomen and then pull the upper abdomen in.

Knees: Relax the knees and bend them slightly.

Feet: Stand with the feet shoulder width apart and the weight evenly distributed. Point the toes in slightly.

Remember:

The main point to remember about the standing position is to keep the upper body relaxed and to concentrate on the lower Dan Tian (lower belly) or, if that is uncomfortable, the soles of your feet. All arm movements should be made using the minimum amount of effort.

If you become unable to relax in the standing position, it is better to bring the exercise to an end and assume another posture in which you are able to relax completely.

The earth's energy, the life force, rises from the bottoms of your feet to the top of your head.

sleeping posture

You should lie on your right side (not on the front or back) and keep the right leg slightly bent (figure 2-5). Rest the left leg on the right leg with the knee bent. The right hand supports the head in such a way that the hand encircles the ear and keeps it open. The upper arm can rest either on the side or folded so that the closed fist rests over the navel.

While falling asleep, concentrate the mind on the lower Dan Tian and let the breathing be as relaxed as possible.

Remember:

One third of your life is spent in sleep. Sleeping the right way is very important.

HOW TO BREATHE

We can go without food and water for many days, yet if we stop breathing for even thirty seconds we quickly realize that we cannot do without air for even a short while. Through bad habits or ignorance, the majority of people breathe very shallow breaths, using only about one third of their lung capacity.

When breathing one usually does not expand and contract the lungs to their full capacity, only the upper sections dilate and shrink, while the lower sections remain virtually unmoving. Since a full supply of oxygen cannot be breathed in, nor all the carbon dioxide breathed out, the blood cannot be completely purified. This bad habit opens the door for any number of illnesses. This is the harmful effect of unnatural breathing.

Natural breathing, also called natural abdominal breathing, is comprised of an inhalation and exhalation that start from the lower belly or lower Dan Tian. Regulating the breath under controlled conditions will enable you to drive your breath downward to the lower abdomen, activating the internal energy held there. This in turn activates the energy so that it will force up and rise as you inhale. When you exhale the diaphragm will relax, taking the pressure off the lower abdomen, and allowing the internal energy to sink back to it. When you inhale, as the air enters, the chest will already be relaxed and the belly will expand. During the inhalation, the huiyin (perineum, figure 2-6) is relaxed. When exhaling the belly should contract and push the diaphragm up to the lungs, forcing out all the impure air. During the exhalation, the huiyin is contracted, or pulled up, maximizing the expulsion of impure air. It is therefore necessary that the respiratory function that expands and contracts the lungs should

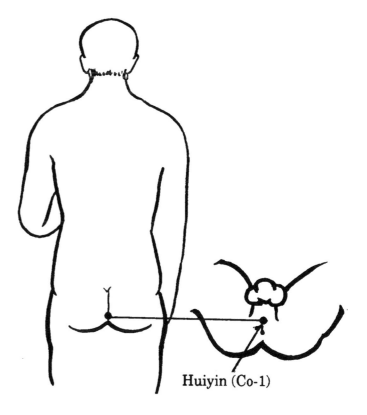

Huiyin (Co-1)

figure 2-6

harmonize with the movements of the belly and diaphragm, thus ensuring free circulation of the blood. This method of breathing should be followed at all times, whether walking, sitting, standing, or reclining. Regular practice of this method will re-train your normal breathing so that healthy, diaphragmatic breathing will become natural and automatic for you.

A short pause should occur naturally and effortlessly after each inhalation and exhalation. You should never force or strain yourself to stop between breaths. There is no need to try and reduce your respiration rate intentionally, just breathe in a relaxed and comfortable way, keeping your breath calm, steady, and silent.

Remember:

One must concentrate on the movements of the lower abdomen. In abdominal breathing the diaphragm is pushed down with every inhalation, causing the lower abdomen to expand, and with every exhalation the diaphragm is pushed up causing the lower abdomen to contract.

Breathing must remain natural and unrestrained.

Moving the abdominal muscles in and out in an intentional and mechanical function will not do.

The upper abdomen should remain motionless, only the lower abdomen should be moving.

POSITION OF THE TONGUE

Relax your tongue and find a position that is comfortable for you.

The spot on the center of the roof of the mouth where the tongue touches is called the Tien Tzie (heavenly pond) or Lung Chuan (Dragon spring)

The purpose of touching the incisor gum with the tongue is to stimulate the secretion of saliva.

Concentrating on raising and

lowering the tongue in time with your breathing will help to keep your mind from becoming distracted by thoughts, thus helping it relax. The up and down motion also stimulates the cerebrum, the part of the brain associated with the digestive organs. This stimulation causes an increase in the excretion of saliva. In Chinese meditation this is called Da Qiao, or building the bridge, because it connects Du Mai and Ren Mai, the two main energy channels in the body.

Remember:

Swallow the saliva. As you swallow the saliva let your mind follow it down to your lower abdomen.

MENTAL ATTITUDE

In Qigong, what one needs to watch is one's own mind. If any emotion, motivation, or thought arises to disturb your peace of mind, do not struggle with it. Do not try to force such thoughts out of your mind. Simply release them and watch as they depart. Detach yourself; be a spectator to the thinking process, not a participant. Concentration of thought is like riding an obstinate mule. Like the mule, a thought will continually take a direction entirely its own. Every time you the rider become aware that your mule, or thought, is straying, you must forcibly turn its head back toward the right path.

The mind affects the body, and the body affects the mind. Qigong makes use of this body/mind relationship. An individual must attempt to concentrate his or her entire mind on the exercises. The mind has to be obedient if you are going to be successful. You have to control, train, and teach it to concentrate on each individual task, whatever it may be, giving it your wholehearted attention. Allow no other thoughts to enter your mind while you are occupied with the task at hand.

Quiet is basic to taking care of the body and it is the foundation of Qigong. When taking care of the body, health and longevity are most easily developed in a state of quiet. During Qigong, one becomes mentally quieter and thinking becomes slower, so the burden on the heart is decreased. If one can attain the state of forgetting one's own body, or remaining quiet without taking mental action, there will be a moment when suddenly all tension is gone, and the mind and body are loose and at ease.

Be patient with your practice and yourself. No one can become an efficient musician in three months or ten easy lessons. Yet most of us expect to win life's best prizes after practicing only a short time, or expending little effort. We become despondent when we fail to realize immediate, significantly recognizable, improvements.

Remember:

Without eagerness or a spirit to learn, learning will be difficult. The secret of learning is joyfulness, fun, and delight.

Patience and indifference to repeated failure are essential in obtaining final success in Qigong.

Do not worry about tomorrow. Tomorrow will take care of itself. Happiness and a calm state of mind are signs of spiritual progress.

CHAPTER 3
GENERAL GUIDELINES FOR PRACTICING

PREPARATION

Relax before doing the exercises. Always allow a short time period before doing Qigong to relax and put the cares of life away. Put yourself in a happy carefree mood, listen to some pleasant music, or visualize a pleasant scene in your mind.

Dress warmly enough so as not to be chilled. Wear loose fitting clothes and loosen your belt. Remove your watch and glasses, undo your shoelaces or remove your shoes.

Drink enough water before practicing so that you will not be thirsty during your practice time.

Go to the restroom if necessary before beginning to practice.

WHERE TO PRACTICE

Choose a quiet spot. Later on you will be able to practice almost anywhere, but for now, you need to eliminate distractions in order to develop your concentration and to be able to relax your body.

Practicing indoors: There should be circulation of fresh air, however you should avoid drafts, especially during the cold winter months because the body usually warms up and sweats a little during Qigong practice. Exposure to a cold draft could give you a cold.

If at all possible do the exercises outside where there is grass, fresh air, trees and flowers.

WHEN TO PRACTICE

The best time to practice Qigong is when you are the happiest, the most relaxed, and in surroundings that are relatively calm and quiet.

If at all possible you should practice once in the morning and once before going to bed.

We spend a lot of time each day just waiting. You can turn that time into practice time.

One should practice for an extended period on the evening or night of the new or full moon day, or at dawn of the following morning. The spiritual potency of these two phases of sun and moon were recognized by almost all ancient sages and seers.

Remember:

The more and the longer you practice, the greater the benefit to you.

WHEN NOT TO PRACTICE

In the beginning, a slight giddiness or discomfort might be felt. At first, when one of the body's organs begins to be used in an unaccustomed way, that organ will naturally resist the unusual activity that is being imposed upon it. If actual pain, distress, a sense of suffocation, or any other abnormal symptoms occur, the exercise should be stopped at once. The student should carefully review the method prescribed to determine whether or not they are practicing it absolutely correctly, because these symptoms will appear only due to either a misunderstanding of the prescribed method, or an organic disease of the organ.

For men only, do not meditate 24 hours before and/or after sex.

Never practice when excited, irritated, or anxious: The benefits of Qigong will not be had because you will not be able to concentrate your mind and will not be able to relax properly. Wait until you are less agitated.

Women should not concentrate on the lower Dan Tian during their menstrual period.

Never practice right after eating. Wait at least one hour. The expanded condition of a full stomach will make it difficult to breathe deeply.

Do not practice when excessively fatigued. The natural thing for the body to do when fatigued and in a calm state is to fall asleep.

Conditions under which Qigong practice is not recommended:

• All diseases in the acute stages

• Retinal bleeding

• Severe bronchitis

• Just after childbirth

• Mental illnesses

Remember:

If you are experiencing pain, discontinue the practice session and try again another day. If the pain continues, contact an experienced Qigong teacher.

How Much to Practice

Beginners: The length should be kept under 30 minutes.

In principle, the longer a meditation lasts the better the result. However, meditation should be natural and the practitioner should avoid straining himself to lengthen the duration.

The amount of time necessary for each person will depend on the individual's physical condition as well as his or her circumstances, such as work schedule and available free time. Those who have serious physical problems and truly wish to improve their condition will want to practice more often (three to six times a day).

NORMAL EFFECTS OF PRACTICING

Yawning, burping, or passing gas, are common reactions that may occur during, or slightly after, Qigong practice. They are part of the process of releasing trapped bad breath, gas, and hot energy from the digestive system. As you inhale, you take cool fresh life force into the esophagus and breath it into the organs. Exhaling while pronouncing the correct sound creates an exchange of energy, bringing the good energy to the organ and forcing out the waste energy.

Some people will experience moving of gas, or loose or very bad smelling bowel movements that are indications of the ongoing detoxification process.

While doing the breathing exercises one may become acutely aware of the beating of his or her heart, not as an excited throbbing, but as a gentle pulsation. This is a natural consequence of the heightened attention being bestowed on the breathing, it need cause no alarm.

Those whose strength and Qi are relatively abundant often experience a swelling sensation or slight stimulation at the top of the nose and at the central point between the eyebrows.

Some people experience an increase in their sexual drive due to the increase in their energy levels. Sexual activity greatly excites the central nervous system and a substantial amount of physical energy is needed to restore the energy lost during ejaculation. Therefore, sexual activity can have a negative influence on the recovery of health. Ancient Qigong masters forbade their students any sexual activities for the first four months of practice. The reason for this was to save and conserve the vital energy (see Editor's Note).

Many people experience involuntary movements during their practice. These movements can vary from small shaking movements to large thrashing movements of the entire body. If these movements occur you should allow them to take place, neither trying to encourage or discourage them. If the movements cause excessive discomfort, concentrate on the soles of the feet rather than the lower Dan Tian. These movements are considered to be a sign of progress.

Increasing the metabolism tends to make the skin softer and smoother. Some people may experience their skin clearing up, even the disappearance of scars and blemishes. Others who practice regularly may experience improvements in their overall sense of well being. Decreases in fatigue, sluggishness, headaches, bronchial complaints such as wheeziness, and so on are quite common. Lack of oxygen places undue stress on the heart and creates many circulatory problems that in turn affect the tissues, bones, glands, organs, and the entire nervous system.

Living in our urban society can subject us to a lifetime full of physical and emotional stresses such as overcrowding, pollution, radiation, junk food, chemical additives, anxiety, loneliness, drug and alcohol abuse, or sudden and overly vigorous exercise. Together these stresses produce tension that blocks the free passage of energy flow in the body causing the organs to overheat. Continued overheating causes the organs to contract and harden. This impairs their ability to function and illnesses result.

Regular Qigong practice helps a person to maintain health, slow down the aging process, live without illness and pain, and even to die peacefully, without bother to family or friends.

ABNORMAL EFFECTS OF PRACTICING

Exhaustion: If your posture is unnatural, or if you remain in the same position for a long time, certain muscles may become strained or fatigued. This can cause you to feel exhausted and weak all over. To avoid this, you should make sure that the posture is comfortable and that your body is relaxed.

Shortness of Breath: Shortness of breath is usually caused by pushing the chest too far forward, bending too far forward at the waist, holding the breath, or trying to breathe too deeply. If you experience shortness of breath, relax your entire body, make sure that your posture is correct, and breathe without straining your diaphragm.

Abdominal Pain and Discomfort: This is usually caused by forcing your breathing to be too deep, or by making your abdominal wall expand and contract unnaturally.

Dizziness and Headaches: If these occur, you should make sure that your tongue stays in touch with the roof of your mouth during inhalation, while at the same time shifting your concentration from your lower Dan Tian to the soles of your feet until the symptoms pass.

Menstrual Problems: For some women, practicing Qigong may influence the menstrual cycle. Qigong may be practiced during this time as long as there are no changes to the length of the menstrual period or the quality of the menstrual flow. If either of these symptoms occurs, the woman must stop concentrating on her lower Dan Tian and switch her focus to the soles of her feet. Concentrating on the lower Dan Tian during the menstrual cycle tends to increase menstrual flow. If either the menstrual flow lengthens or the quantity of the flow increases, and changing the point of concentration does not help, discontinue practice until the period is over.

Falling Asleep: Some people become drowsy, and others may fall asleep, when practicing Qigong, especially in the lying down posture. Although this may be a result of the body being in a complete state of relaxation, the benefits of the Qigong are lost. To keep from falling asleep, practice with your eyes open.

CHAPTER 4
SIX HEALING SOUNDS QIGONG

BASIC PRINCIPLES

Controlling the breath is one of the most important aspects of Six Healing Sounds Qigong. Through proper breathing, the organs of the body are strengthened and their functions are improved. Inhalation brings nourishment into the body and assists blood circulation and organ function. Exhalation, using the correct sound, serves to cleanse the body of harmful elements and wastes, and to speed up the heat exchange through the digestive system.

The resting period in between each sound is very important. It is the time in which you are becoming in touch with, and more aware of, the organs.

Remember:

The abdomen expands during inhalation and contracts during exhalation.

The huiyin (perineum) relaxes with the inhalation, and contracts (pulls up) with the exhalation.

The tongue touches the roof of the mouth just behind the front teeth during inhalation, and drops to the floor of the mouth during exhalation.

All sounds are made slowly and evenly

Perform each exercise from 6 to 12 times.

Do not practice these exercises within 1 hour of eating, before or after a meal.

The Daoist system of Qigong gives each organ different characteristics, the list in the next column is an example of the descriptions that you will find for each organ system:

- One of the five elements in nature (metal, water, wood, fire or earth).

- A season of the year (autumn, winter, spring, summer, or late summer) that is determined by which season the organ is dominant or working the hardest.

- A color, a quality in nature, a direction, a planet.

- An emotion (joy, anger, etc.)

- A time of day based on the time of the day the Qi is flowing in that meridian.

You will find the characteristics for each organ at the beginning of each section.

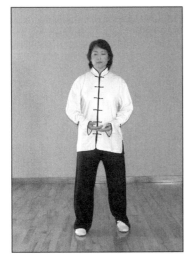

figure 4-1

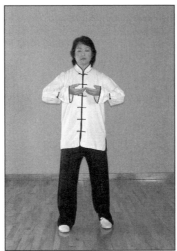

figure 4-2

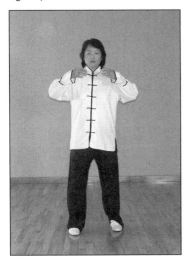

figure 4-3

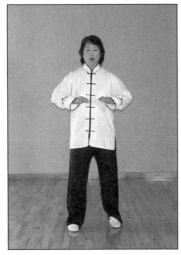

figure 4-4

THE SIX HEALING SOUNDS

transitional movements

These are the "transitional movements" that are to be done before and after each exercise session, and following the completion of each of the organ sets within the session.

These movements are done between ALL exercises. For example, if you have finished the Heart exercise and you are going to go on to another exercise, do these movements before continuing to the next exercise.

When you are finished with your Six Healing Sounds set, perform these movements six times, remain still for a minute or two, and then resume your normal activities.

Begin by breathing in slowly using the diaphragm. At the same time bring the hands slowly up to the chest (figures 4-1 and 4-2). At this point you have inhaled fully, your lower Dan Tian has expanded and is full of air. Turn your palms over, so they are facing down (figure 4-3). Now begin to exhale slowly using the sound "CAW." Keep the mind centered on the lower Dan Tian. Bring in the abdomen, at the same time lower the hands slowly and in time with the exhalation of air (figure 4-4). Now turn the palms over and begin the exercise again.

Remember:

Relax the entire body.

The mind and hands guide the air in and out and are in harmony with the breathing.

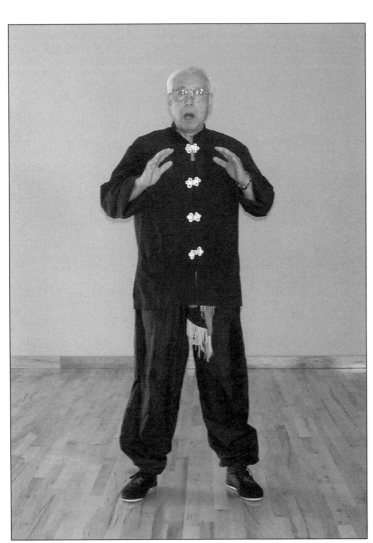

heart exercise

Organ: Heart

Sound: "CAW"

Function: Controls all of the other organs because it controls the blood circulation

Chinese function: Stores the spirit and controls mental and emotional activities. Spirit, memory, thinking, and sleep are all dominated by the heart.

Associated organ: Small intestine

Direction: South

Element: Fire

Season; Summer

Planet: Mars

Taste: Bitter

Color: Red

Body Part: Tongue

Sense: Speech, taste

Positive Emotions: Joy, laughter

Negative Emotions: Violence, cruelty

Pronouncing the Sound: The "CAW" sound is made by opening the mouth the width of two fingers with the tongue down and behind the lower teeth (figure 4-5). The sound is made by bringing the abdomen in and allowing the exhaling air to produce the sound. The sound should be slow and even. Use the mind to control the air.

Remember: When exhaling, the big toes and the thumbs are pushed down.

figure 4-5

HEART MOVEMENTS

Inhale:

Begin by inhaling slowly. The mind is guiding the breath. Slowly raise the hands with the palms up to a level slightly higher than the waist (figures 4-6 and 4-7). At this point you have inhaled fully and your abdomen has expanded.

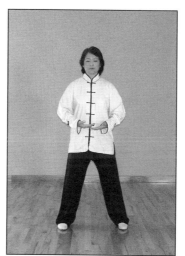

figure 4-6

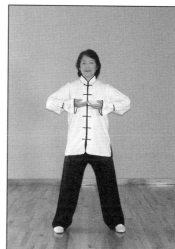

figure 4-7

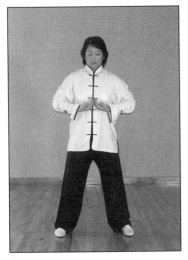

figure 4-8

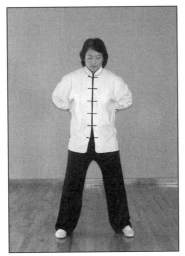

figure 4-9

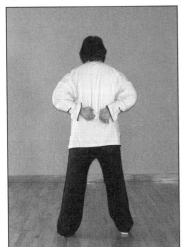

figure 4-10

Hold your breath while turning the palms so that the palms are facing up, the backs of the hand touching (figure 4-8).

Exhale: (sound is "CAW")

Exhale as you move the hands to the small of your back and massage the kidneys (figures 4-9 and 4-10).

When you have reached the small of the back, bring your hands out to the sides, palms facing up (figure 4-11), until the backs of the hands touch (figure 4-12). Putting pressure on the Hapku points improves circulation and breathing, reduces or relieves headaches, and relaxes nerves. It clears the large intestine meridian, giving a good foundation for the Qi Life Cycle. Connect the Hapku points and press the hands gently together. (figure 4-13). The abdomen should now be in and all of the air exhaled from the body.

Remember: The entire body should be relaxed.

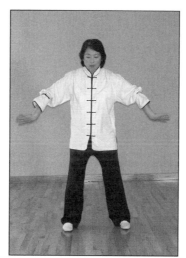

figure 4-11   figure 4-12

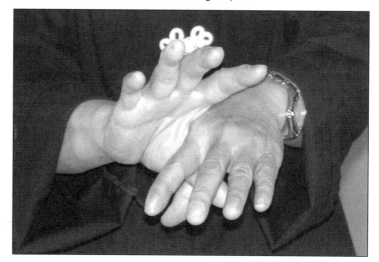

figure 4-13

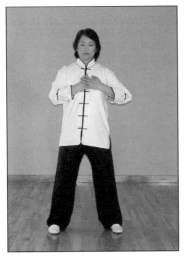

figure 4-14

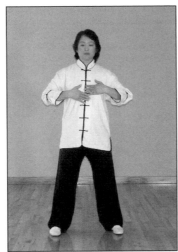

figure 4-15

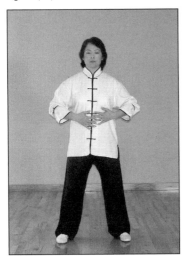

figure 4-16

Inhale:

Inhale while separating and making two small circles with the hands, palms facing out and in front of you. Bring the hands to the chest with the palms facing, and gently touching, the body (figure 4-14).

The abdomen is now fully expanded.

Hold Your Breath:

Slowly bring the hands down in front of you, gently touching your body until your hands are in front of your lower abdomen (figures 4-15 to 4-16).

Raise your hands with the palms facing up to waist level (figure 4-17).

Remember:

Keep the entire body relaxed.

Exhale (sound is "CAW")

Exhale slowly, while turning the hands with the palms facing forward. Push the hands forward, outward, and up (figures 4-18 to 4-19). Visualize them pushing an object of great weight. Relax and do not tense any muscles.

Remember:

The "CAW" sound is slow and even, and comes from the diaphragm.

Inhale:

Inhale slowly while bringing the hands (palms in) slowly to the upper chest area. At this time the abdomen should be extended and the body full of air (figure 4-20).

While holding your breath slowly lower your hands with the palms facing and gently touching the body (figures 4-21 and 4-22). As the hands are moving downward the mind is visualizing the Qi being pushed down to the lower Dan Tian (lower abdomen). Slowly exhale. Lower the hands to the lower abdomen, bring them up to waist level and begin the entire sequence again.

Remember:

During exhalation the big toes and the thumbs are gently pushed down.

This entire sequence is one repetition and should be performed once or twice, depending on how you are feeling and the amount of available time.

At the end of heart exercise, the hands return to the Lower Dan Tian, ladies right hand on the bottom left hand on top, men left hand on the bottom right hand on top.

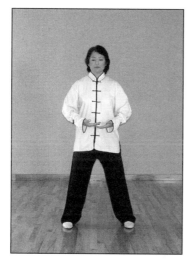

figure 4-17

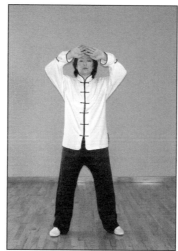

figure 4-18

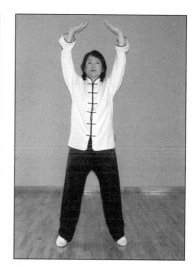

figure 4-19

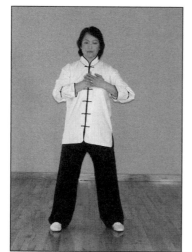

figure 4-20

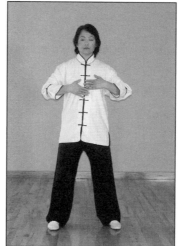

figure 4-21

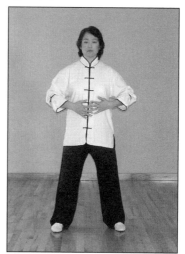

figure 4-22

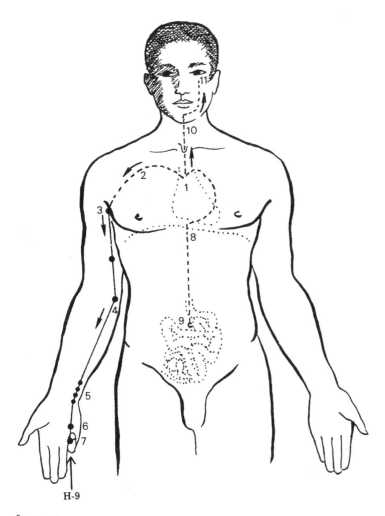

H-9

figure 4-23

HEART MERIDIAN

Heart Meridian: Yin
Number of points on each
side of the body: 9
Beginning at the base of the
armpit and traveling down the
inner side of the arm to the base
of the smallest finger (figure 4-
23).
Time of day: II A.M.–I A.M.
Disorders treated on the heart
meridian: Emotional problems,
anxiety, insomnia, and heart
disorders.
*Perform the Transitional
Movements (figures 4-1 to
4-4) before proceeding to
the next organ set or
ending the session.*

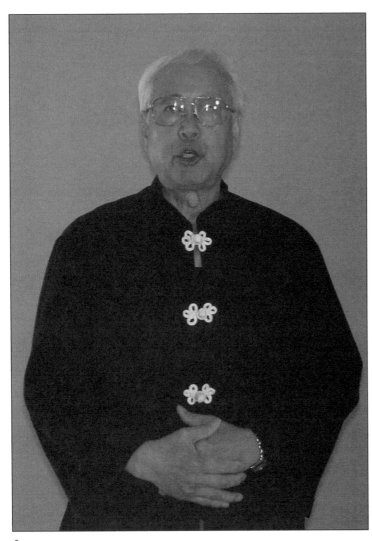

figure 4-24

liver exercise

Organ: Liver

Sound: "SHHH"

Function: Stores blood and regulates the volume of blood circulating.

Chinese Function: Stores the soul and regulates the flow of vital energy.

Associated Organ: Gall bladder

Direction: East

Element: Wood

Season: Spring

Planet: Jupiter

Taste: Sour

Color: Green

Sense: Sight

Body Part: Eyes

Positive Emotions: Kindness

Negative Emotions: Anger

Pronouncing the Sound: The "SHHH" sound is made as if one were trying to quiet a child (figure 4-24). The tongue is down, the teeth are together, and the lips are parted. When made correctly, this sound affects the Renzhong point (figure 4-25) beneath the nose.

LIVER MOVEMENTS

Remember:

Keep the shoulders relaxed as you push in with the hands.

The men should have the right hand over the left and the women should have the left over the right hand.

Pronouncing the Sound: "SHHH."

The following "Liver" exercise has five repetitions.

Placement of Hands:

Regardless of gender, left hand on liver (diaphragm) right hand over left. First, inhale slowly through your nose, proceed with the (long) exhale of "SHHH" (figure 4-26) Now, inhale slowly through the nose, keeping the mouth closed (figure 4-27). Remember, in order to control the lower Dan Tian, the stomach must tighten during exhalation and fill with air during inhalation.

Perform the Transitional Movements (figures 4-1 to 4-4) before proceeding to the next organ set or ending the session.

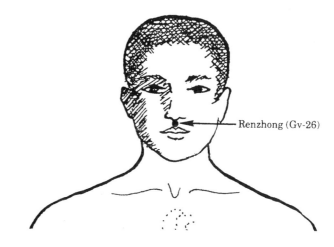

Renzhong (Gv-26)

figure 4-25

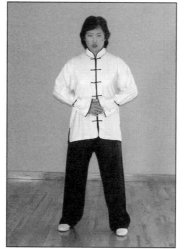

figure 4-26

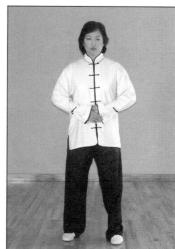

figure 4-27

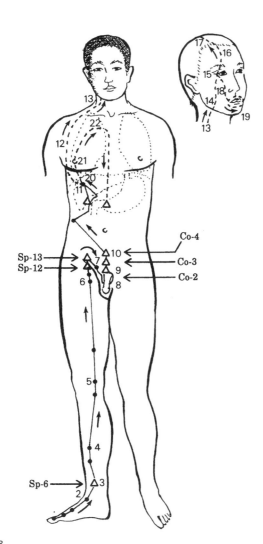

figure 4-28

LIVER MERIDIAN

Liver Meridian: Yin

Number of points on each side of the body: 14

Beginning at the base of the nail on the big toe, it then travels up the inside of the legs and thighs and ends at a point near the nipples (figure 4-28).

Time of day: 1 A.M.–3 A.M.

Disorders involved with the liver meridian: Diabetes, arthritis, uterine disorders, colds, and liver problems.

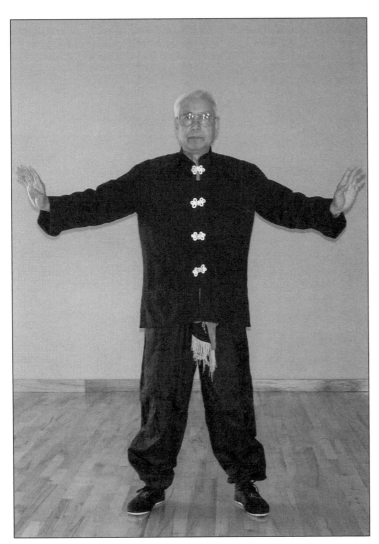

figure 4-29

lung exercise

Organ: Lungs

Sound: "SSSS"

Function: Essential organs of
respiration: The lungs inhale
fresh air to supply the body's
functions and exhale waste air.

Chinese Function: To activate the
flow of vital energy (Qi).

Associated Organ: Large Intestine

Direction: West

Element: Metal

Season: Autumn

Planet: Venus

Taste: Pungent

Color: White

Senses: Smell

Body Part: Skin, nose.

Positive Emotions: Courage

Negative Emotion: Anxiety

Pronouncing the Sound: The sound
"SSS" is made by closing the jaw
so that the teeth meet gently, part
the lips slightly, draw the corners
of the mouth back and allow the
breath to escape through the
spaces between the teeth (figure
4-29). The sound is similar to
the sound you hear when using a
bicycle pump as it puts the air
into the tire, or the hissing of a
snake.

Remember:

The corners of the mouth are
pulled back during exhalation.

LUNG MOVEMENTS

Pronouncing the Sound:
"SSS."

Inhale: Tongue up

Exhale: Tongue down.

Inhale until hands are in the position of figure 4-30, begin to exhale "SSS" until arms are fully extended (figures 4-31 and 4-33). Bringing your hands back down and in as shown in figures 4-34 to 4-36.

Repeat this exercise five times.

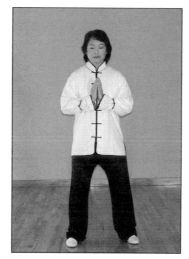

figure 4-30

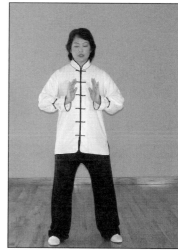

figure 4-31

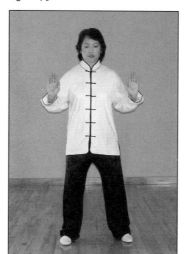

figure 4-32

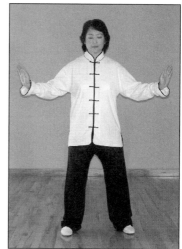

figure 4-33

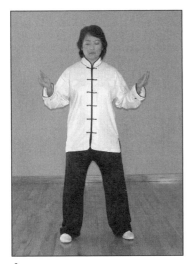

figure 4-34

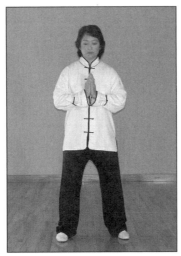

figure 4-35

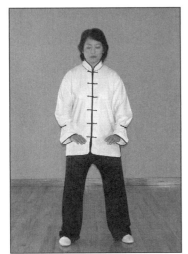

figure 4-36

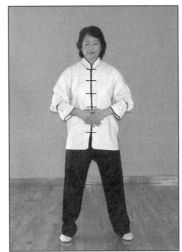

figure 4-37

To end this set, return hands to Lower Dan Tian (figure 4-37), ladies right hand on the bottom left hand on top, men left hand on the bottom right hand on top.

Now, go back and perform your Movements to be Done Between sets 6 times.

Perform the Transitional Movements (figures 4-1 to 4-4) before proceeding to the next organ set or ending the session.

LUNG MERIDIANS

Lung Meridian: Yin

Number of points on each side of the body: 11

Beginning near the armpit, between the second and third ribs, and runs along the upper and lower arms ending on the inside of the thumb at the root of the nail (figure 4-38).

Time of Day: 3 A.M.–5 A.M.

Disorders treated on the lung meridian: Respiratory problems, asthma, bronchitis, coughing, throat disorders, anxiety, and restlessness.

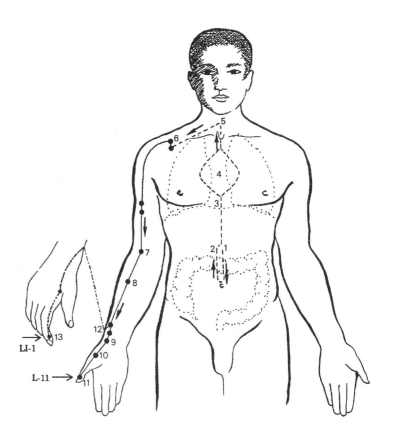

figure 4-38

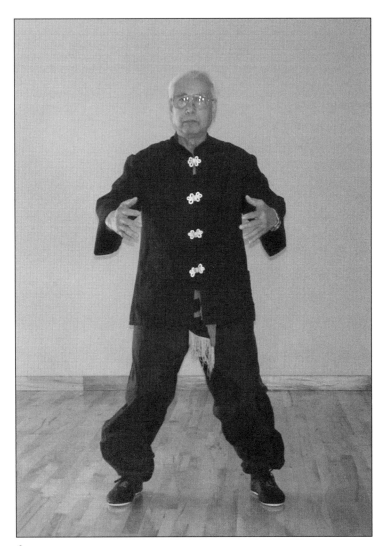

kidney exercise

Organ: Kidneys

Sound: "CHUEE"

Function: Removes toxic materials from the blood.

Chinese Function: To store essence of life that is inherited and acquired from food.

Associated Organ: Bladder

Direction: North

Element: Water

Season: Winter

Planet: Mercury

Taste: Salty

Color: Black

Body Parts: Ears

Sense: Hearing

Positive Emotions: Gentleness

Negative Emotions: Fear

Pronouncing the Sound: The sound "CHUEE." The sound is made by bringing the abdomen in and letting the exhaling air make the sound. The "CHU" sound should be short and sharp, and the "EE" should be long, slow, and even.

Remember: The body should be relaxed. The breathing should be slow and even (figure 4-39).

figure 4-39

Kidney Movements

Inhale:

Begin by inhaling slowly, and raising the hands with the palms up to a level slightly higher than your waist (figure 4-40). At this point you have inhaled fully and your abdomen has expanded.

Hold Your Breath:

Turn the hands so the palms are facing out, the back of the hand is touching the side of the body. Move the hands to the small of your back, massaging the kidneys, rubbing up and down six times (figures 4-41 and 4-42). When you have reached the small of the back, bring your hands out and up to the front of your body until the backs of the hands touch at chest level (figures 4-43 and 4-44). The abdomen is still expanded.

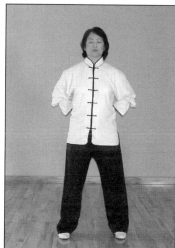

figure 4-40

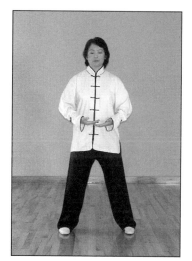

figure 4-41

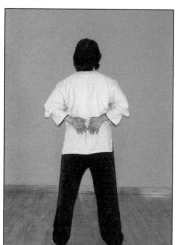

figure 4-42

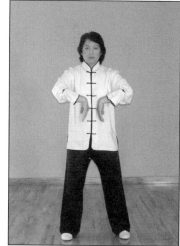

figure 4-43

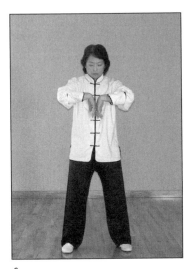

figure 4-44

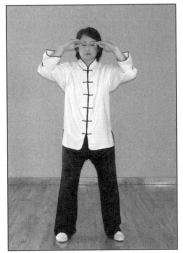

figure 4-45

Exhale: (sound is "CHUEE")
Exhale using the diaphragm to force the air out and to pronounce the sound. As you exhale, the hands move apart and the palms move up and face each other (figure 4-45). The hands and arms continue outward until they are at shoulder level and shoulder width apart (figure 4-46). The hands and arms now look as if they are holding a large ball).

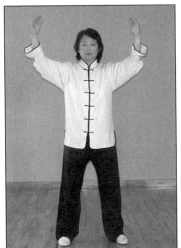

figure 4-46

Now slowly bend the knees and lower the body as if you were going to sit on a small stool. The thighs should be parallel to the floor, the upper body leaning forward, the arms still shoulder width apart (figures 4-47 to 4-49). The abdomen should be in and all of the air expelled.

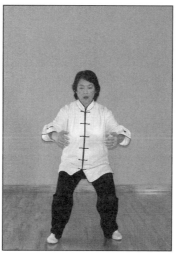

figure 4-47

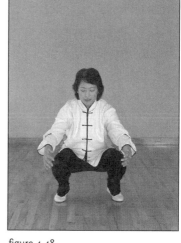

figure 4-48

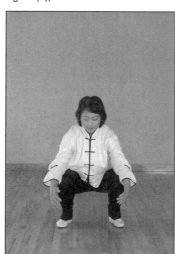

figure 4-49

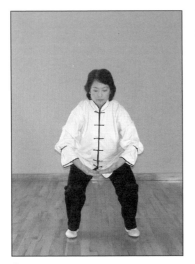

figure 4-50

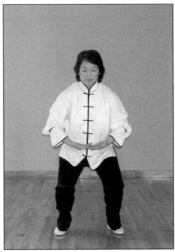

figure 4-51

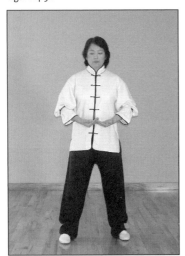

figure 4-52

Inhale:

Inhale slowly, bringing the hands together (figure 4-50). Slowly begin to stand up, raising the hands and visualizing them lifting a great weight (figure 4-51). Continue until the hands reach waist level. The abdomen is now extended and full of air.(figure 4-52)

Exhale: Repeat this entire sequence once or twice, depending on how you are feeling and the amount of available time.

Return hands to Lower Dan Tian, ladies right hand on the bottom left hand on top, men left hand on the bottom right hand on top.

Perform the Transitional Movements (figures 4-1 to 4-4) before proceeding to the next organ set or ending the session.

Kidney Meridian

Kidney meridian: Yin
Number of points on each side of the body: 27

Beginning on the sole of the foot, traveling up the inside of the leg to the center of the body, and ending just below the collarbone, between the clavicle and the first rib (figure 4-53).

Time of Day: 5 P.M.–7 P.M.

Disorders involved with this meridian: Gastritis, liver infections, hernia, eye disorders, vomiting.

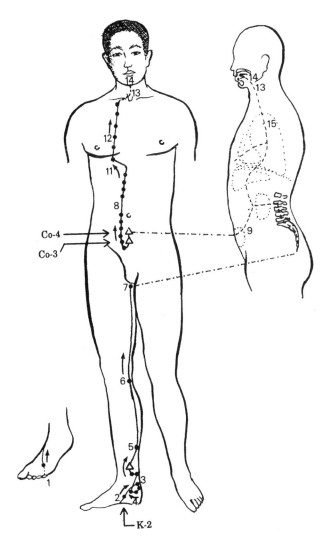

figure 4-53

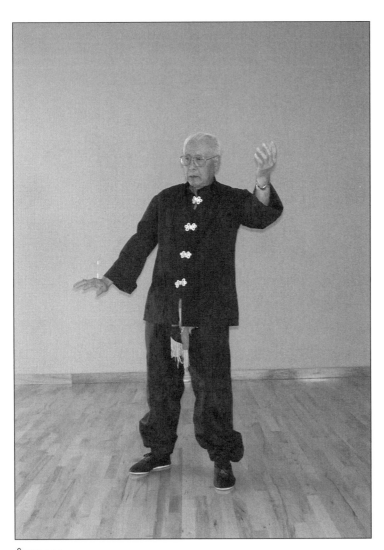

figure 4-54

stomach/spleen exercise

Organ: Stomach

Sound: "WHO" Aspirated

Function: The principle organ of digestion, the stomach receives and decomposes food.

Associated organ: Spleen

Chinese Function: The stomach and spleen are like warehouses where a person's food and essences are stored. From *The Yellow Emperor's Classic of Medicine* translated by Maoshin Ni, Ph.D.

Direction: Center

Element: Earth

Season: Indian Summer

Planet: Saturn

Taste: Neutral

Color: Yellow

Body Part: Mouth

Sense: Taste

Positive Emotions: Compassion

Negative Emotions: Worry

Pronouncing the Sound: The sound "WHO" is slightly aspirated ("HWHO"), and made by rounding the mouth and visualizing blowing out a candle (figure 4-54). The sound is made by bringing the abdomen in slowly and allowing the exhaling air to make the sound. The sound is slow and even.

Remember: Relax the entire body. The mind controls the movements, use as little force as possible.

STOMACH MOVEMENTS

Begin by exercising your right side first, right palm over left for men, left palm over right for women (figure 4-55). Slowly raise the right arm while exhaling the sound "Who," and turning palm up slowly as your hand raises over your head (figures 4-56 to 4-58). Left palm will face downward, and you will bring your abdomen in slowly as you exhale.

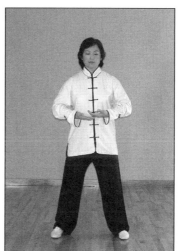

figure 4-55

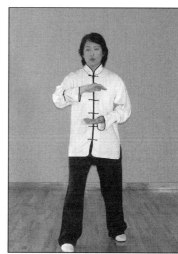

figure 4-56

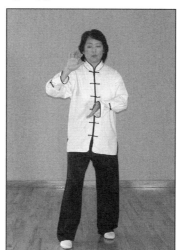

figure 4-57

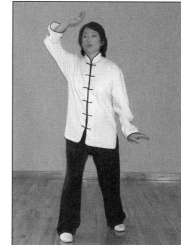

figure 4-58

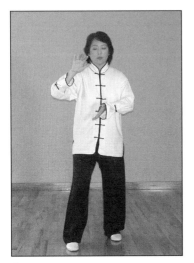

figure 4-59

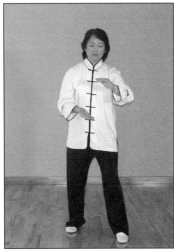

figure 4-60

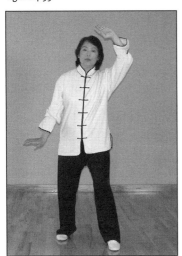

figure 4-61

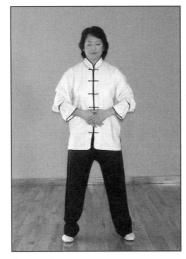

figure 4-62

Now, inhale very slowly through the nose, the air is slowly entering the stomach, bring right hand down slowly (figures 4-59 and 4-60), turn palms and reverse the exercise for the left side, left palm rising slowly over your head, right palm turning to face downward (figures 4-61 and 4-62). Repeat the entire exercise 5 times on each side.

Important: If you have high blood pressure do not raise your hands above your head, move them out in front of your body instead.

Stomach exercise, is done by pronouncing the sound "WHO." The hand follows the sound and the sound follows the breathing.

RIGHT SIDE

Exhale:
Pronouncing the Sound "WHO."
Inhale:
Mouth closed, breathing in through nose slowly, relaxing the body and mind.

Stomach exercise, is done by pronouncing the sound "WHO." The hand follows the sound and the sound follows the breathing.

LEFT SIDE

Exhale.
Pronouncing the Sound: "WHO."
Inhale.
Mouth closed, breathing in through nose slowly, relaxing the body and mind.

Exhale: Repeat this entire sequence once or twice, depending on how you are feeling and the amount of available time.

Return Hands to Lower Dan Tian, ladies right hand on the bottom left hand on top, men left hand on the bottom right hand on top (figure 4-62).

Perform the Transitional Movements (figures 4-1 to 4-4) before proceeding to the next organ set or ending the session.

STOMACH MERIDIAN

Stomach meridian: Yang

Number of points on each side of the body: 45

Beginning just under the eye, moving down the body and legs, and ending at the feet (figure 4-63).

Time of Day: 7 A.M.–9 A.M.

Disorders treated on the stomach meridian: All infections of the abdominal organs, eye disorders, mouth disorders, paralysis, and nervous disorders.

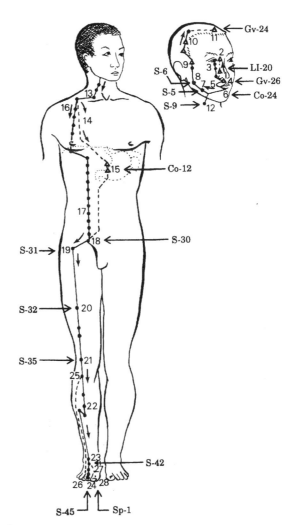

figure 4-63

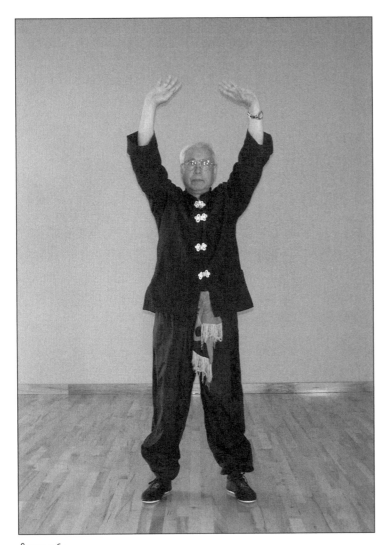

figure 4-64

triple warmer exercise

Organ: Triple warmer or sometimes
referred to as the Triple Heater,
refers to the three energy centers
(the upper, middle, and lower
Dan Tians).

Sound: "SHEEE"

Chinese Function: Balances the
temperature of the three energy
centers.

Element: Internal fire

Season: None

Planet: None

Taste: None

Color: None

Body Part: Chest

Pronouncing the Sound: The sound
"SHEEE" is made with the teeth
slightly apart. The sound is slow
and even (figure 4-64).

Remember:

Keep the shoulders relaxed as
you raise the hands over your
head.

*If you have high blood
pressure do not raise your
hands above your head.
Instead push them out in
front of you at shoulder
level.*

TRIPLE WARMER MOVEMENTS

Pronouncing the Sound: "SHEEE."

Inhale: Slowly through nose, mouth closed.

Exhale: Teeth slightly apart, slowly.

Inhale bringing hands up slowly (figure 4-65), turning palms up then outward (figure 4-66), when you reach figure 4-67 begin to exhale sound "SHEEE" extending arms high (palms up).

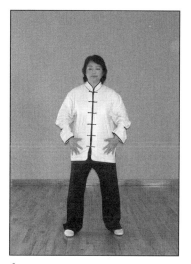

figure 4-65

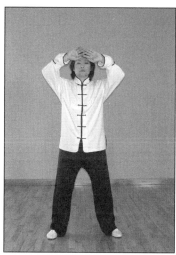

figure 4-66

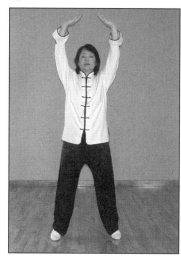

figure 4-67

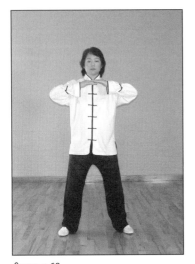

figure 4-68

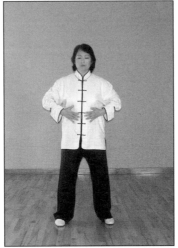

figure 4-69

At figure 4-68 slowly inhale and bring your arms down, continuing through figure 4-69.

As you bring hands down, touch the chest pushing downward. Return Hands to Lower Dan Tian and gently exhale, ladies right hand on the bottom left hand on top, men left hand on the bottom right hand on top (figure 4-70). Repeat this exercise ten times.

Remember to keep shoulders relaxed as you raise your hands over your head.

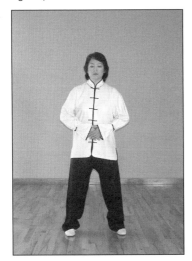

figure 4-70

Triple Warmer Meridians

Triple Warmer Meridian: Yang
   Number of points on each
side of the body: 23
   Beginning at the hand it
travels up the hand and arm to
the head, where it ends near the
eye, under the eyebrow (figure
4-71).
   Time of Day: 9 P.M.–11 P.M.
   Disorders relating to the
Triple Warmer: Constipation,
diabetes, deafness, paralysis and
arthritis.

   *Perform the Transitional
   Movements (figures 4-1 to
   4-4) before ending your
   Six Healing Movements
   session.*

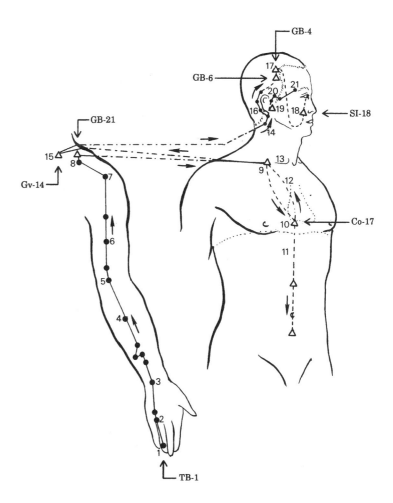

figure 4-71

CHAPTER 5

OTHER QIGONG EXERCISES

GENERAL GUIDELINES

Beginning of Exercises. Breathe in slowly (using the diaphragm) while bringing the hands up to waist level. Bring the hands together. Hold the air in the lower Dan Tian. Rub the hands and palms together (feel the heat in the palms). Bring the hands to the area to be exercised.

Now Do an Exercise.

Remember: Relax, breathe in slowly using the diaphragm, and allow the tongue to touch the roof of the mouth. Let the mind move the hands in unison with the breath.

Ending of Exercises. Exhale slowly using the sound "Caa." Bring the hands down slowly until they are hanging relaxed in front of you.

Remember: Relax, exhale slowly using the Caa sound; tongue is now down and behind the teeth. Let the mind move the hands down in unison with the exhalation of the air.

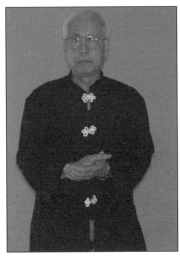

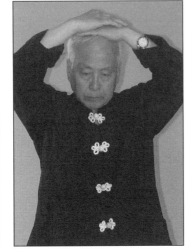

figure 5-1   figure 5-2

HEAD EXERCISE:

scalp rub

Rub hands together, then slowly bring them to the middle of the head (men left hand on bottom and right hand on top, women right hand on bottom and left hand on top) and gently massage the scalp from side to side and from front to back (figures 5-1 and 5-2).

beating the heavenly drum

Rub hands together (figure 5-3), then bring them to the face. Massage the cheeks while moving the hands to the ears. Palms should cover the ears, thumbs placed below the ears. Gently push the hands against the ears causing a suction sensation in the ears (figures 5-4 and 5-5). Now beat the four finger tips on the mid line on the back of the head. Bring the hand down while massaging the neck (figure 5-6).

Remember: Relax the shoulders.

Function: Increases the circulation of blood and Qi in the head area. Helps calm and clear the mind, and also improves the memory. Improves the health of the scalp and helps prevent loss of hair.

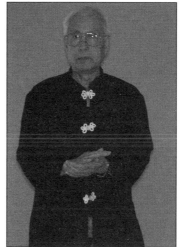

figure 5-3

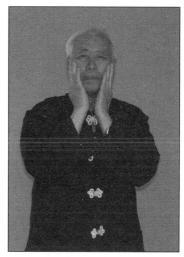

figure 5-4

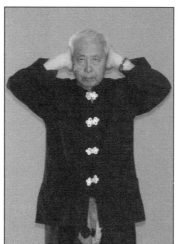

figure 5-5

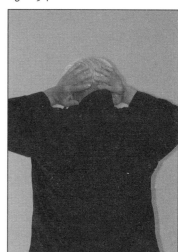

figure 5-6

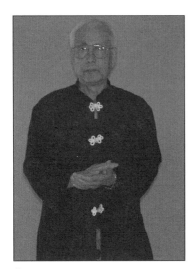

figure 5-7

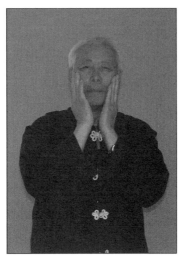

figure 5-8

face and eye rub

First rub hands together (figure 5-7), then bring them to the face. Massage above and below the eyes, close the eyes and gently massage the eyelids (figures 5-8 to 5-9).

Function: Improves circulation in the face and improves the complexion.

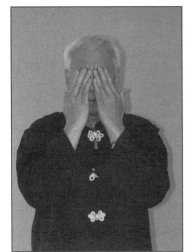

figure 5-9

nose rub

Rub hands together (figure 5-10), then slowly bring them to the side of the nose. Massage both sides of the nose (figure 5-11).

Function: Helps relieve congestion caused by nasal and sinus problems.

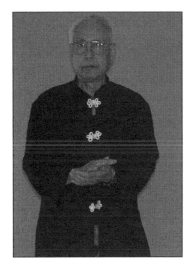
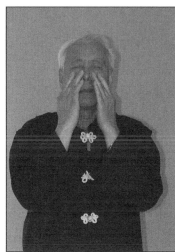

figure 5-10   figure 5-11

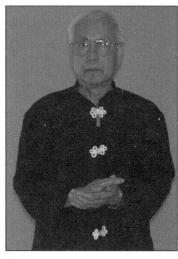

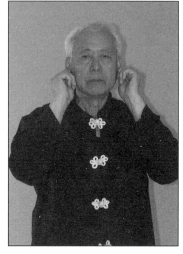

figure 5-12   figure 5-13

ear rub

Rub hands together (figure 5-12), then slowly bring them to the ears. Massage the ears and ear lobes (figure 5-13).

Function: Stimulates the circulatory and respiratory centers in the brain. Effective for headaches.

neck exercises

Rub hands together (figure 5-14), then bring them to the top of the head, with palms facing down (men with right hand over left, women with left hand over right) Slowly lower your head and move it in a clockwise direction while breathing in (figure 5-15). Continue to rotate your head slowly until you reach the halfway point, then begin to exhale slowly continuing in a clockwise direction. Do this six times and then reverse direction and move in a counterclockwise direction.

Function: Relieves tension from the neck and shoulders. Improves circulation in the neck and shoulders. Alleviates dizziness.

Now lower your hands to your side. Gently turn your head first to the right side (figure 5-16) and then to the left side (figure 5-17). Do this ten times on each side .

Then place hands crossed over your shoulder, grabbing and holding. This will eliminate pressure and tight muscles. You will feel your hands pulling downward (figure 5-18).

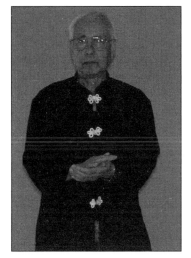

figure 5-14

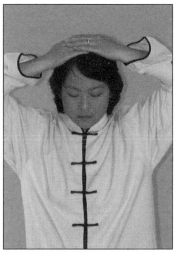

figure 5-15

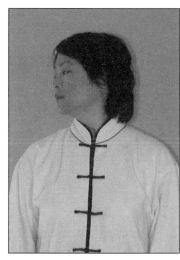

figure 5-16

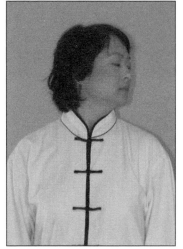

figure 5-17

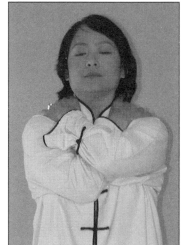

figure 5-18

location of the meridians on the head

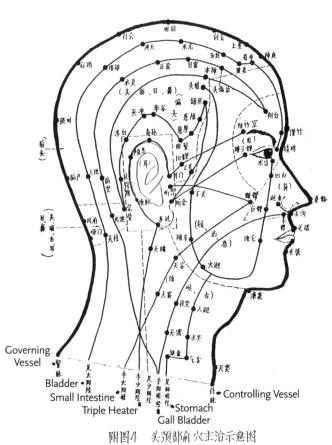

Governing Vessel

Bladder

Small Intestine

Triple Heater

Stomach

Gall Bladder

Controlling Vessel

附图4 头预部俞穴主治示意图

figure 5-19

BODY EXERCISES

shoulder exercise

Inhale slowly through your nose while doing this exercise. From the starting position (figure 5-20), slowly raise the hands and shoulders (figure 5-21). Your shoulders will be up high. Now, you will start to exhale through the mouth bringing hands down slowly. (figure 5-22)

A variation on this exercise would be to use the starting position (figure 5-22). Inhale slowly through your nose while bringing the hands up (figures 5-23 and 5-24). Then exhale through the mouth and move the hands down (figure 5-25).

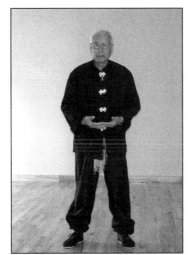

figure 5-20

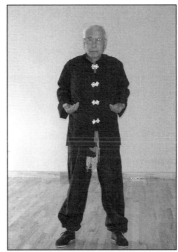

figure 5-21

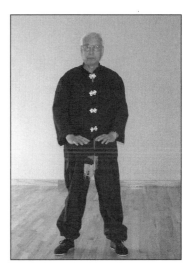

figure 5-22

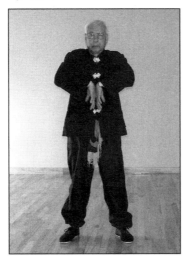

figure 5-23

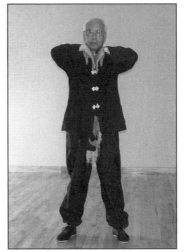

figure 5-24

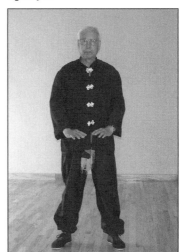

figure 5-25

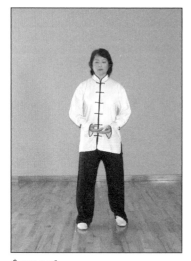

figure 5-26

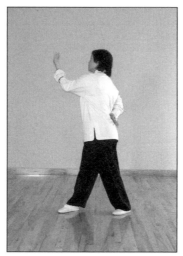

figure 5-27

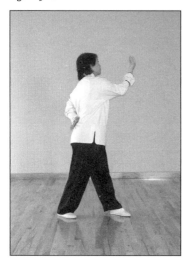

figure 5-28

kidney and shoulder twist (can koon-pak quaw)

The Chinese call this kidney location "Life Door" or Ming-Men. This exercise proves to be excellent for blood circulation, and is actually done by slapping yourself. This exercise requires that the arms hang loosely. The turning of the body generates enough momentum in the arms that they gently 'hit' the kidney and shoulder areas after your torso stops turning.

Feet are positioned about two feet apart (figure 5-26). Slowly inhaling, slap right hand over kidney and twist to the right and slap left hand on shoulder (figure 5-27). Exhaling, twist to the left side and bring left hand down over kidney and proceed to swing right hand on left shoulder (figure 5-28).

Repeat this exercise ten times each side.

kidney exercise

Warm kidneys by first rubbing (massaging) six times. Repeat to rub your buttocks.

Slowly inhale and rotate (figures 5-30 to 5-33), now exhale and rotate to the left side. Note: How long your breath may last will determine how many circles you will make before switching to the other side, for example you might make two circles before you have to inhale. It is very important that your breathing begin with the right side first. The better your breathing becomes the more circles you will make. When you practice this exercise, three parts of your body will circle in unison, ankles, knees, and kidneys.

Repeat this exercise ten times in each direction.

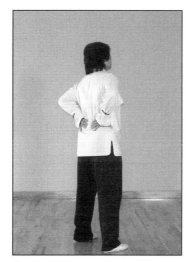
figure 5-30

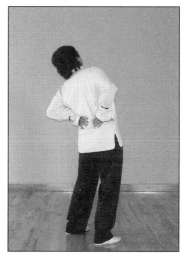
figure 5-31

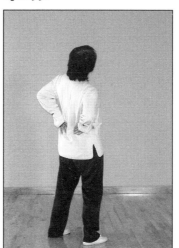
figure 5-32

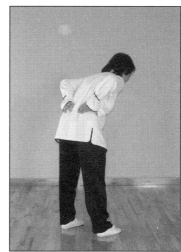
figure 5-33

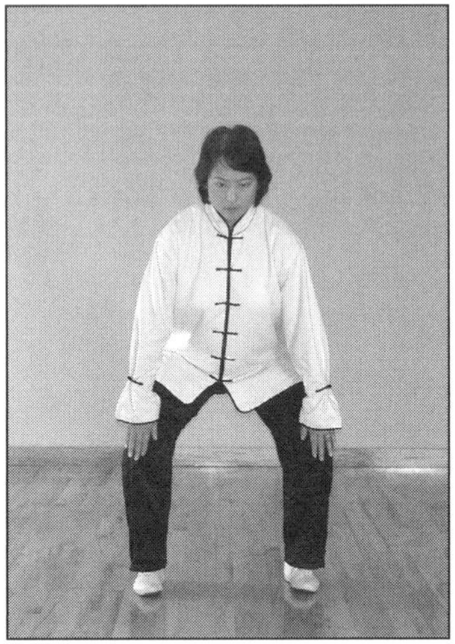

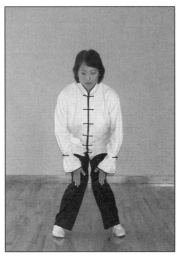

figure 5-34

figure 5-35

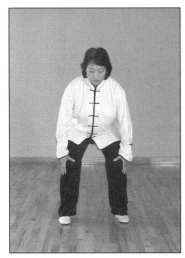

figure 5-36

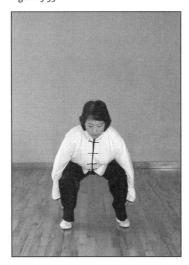

figure 5-37

Knee Exercise

Inhale, push knees outward (figure 5-34). Exhale, push knees inward (figure 5-35). Repeat five times before continuing to the next part.

Place hands on the front of your knees and inhale (figure 5-36). Move hands to the back of knees and exhale as they move down the back of your legs to touch your ankles (figure 5-37). Keeping your hands behind your legs, rise up while inhaling. Next, go down while inhaling. Repeat five times.

dan tian rub

Ladies right hand on the bottom left hand on top (figure 5-38), men left hand on the bottom right hand on top (figure 5-39). Gently circle the hands over and around the navel in a clockwise direction until the area feels warm.

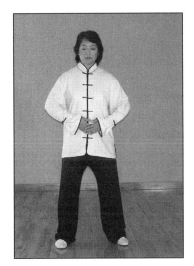

figure 5-38

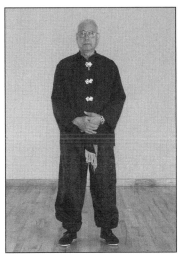

figure 5-39

CHAPTER 6
CIRCULATING ENERGY IN THE MICROCOSMIC ORBIT

ENERGY CENTERS

It is much easier to cultivate your energy if you first understand the major paths of energy circulation in the body. The nervous system in humans is very complex and is capable of directing energy wherever it is needed. The ancient Daoist masters discovered that there are two energy channels that carry an especially strong current.

The first channel (Ren Mai) is called the functional or yin channel. It begins at the base of the trunk, midway between a man's testicles or a woman's vagina and the anus at a point called the perineum, and travels up the front of the body past the sex organ, stomach, heart, and throat, ending at the tip of the tongue (figure 6-1).

The second channel (Du Mai) is called the governor channel or the yang channel (figure 6-2). Du Mai starts in the same place as Ren Mai, but travels up the back of the body. It flows from the perineum upwards into the tailbone (tip of the coccyx) and then up through the spine into the brain, down the middle of the forehead to the roof of the mouth.

The tongue is like a switch that connects these two currents. When it is touched to the roof of the mouth just behind the front teeth, the energy can flow in a circle up the spine and back down the front.

The two channels form a single circuit that the energy loops around. This circulating energy, known as the microcosmic orbit, forms the basis of acupuncture.

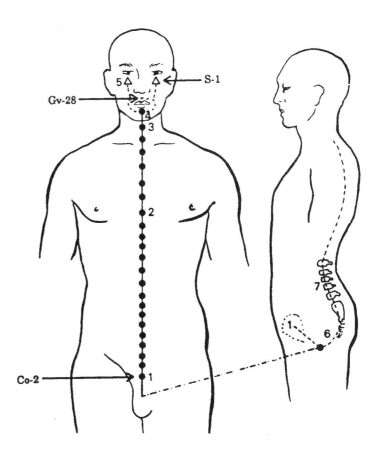

figure 6-1

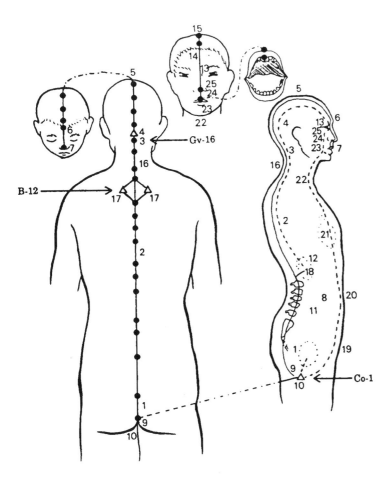

figure 6-2

Basic Principles in Opening Up the Energy Channels

To awaken the energy in the individual points use your inner vision. Direct your vision inwardly to the point you wish to activate, and then concentrate your mind on that point in your body. Do not create a visual image of the energy point in your mind, rather bring your mind down from your head and put it in a specific point in your body, in this example, your navel.

When you concentrate on the navel, focus one and one half inches below the skin. In the beginning, apply pressure on the point with your index finger for one to five minutes, then return your hands to your lap and concentrate on the sensations created by your fingers, pressing again when the point becomes indistinct.

Be sure to direct your inner vision down to your navel when you finish your practice period.

Collecting the energy gathers up the excess Qi in the body and stores it in the navel. It protects your body organs from accumulating too much energy. To do this, concentrate on your navel as you place your right fist there. Rotate your fist 6 times clockwise allowing the circle to grow larger until it is no more than 6 inches in diameter, not higher than the heart nor lower than the pelvis. Then reverse the direction of rotation and rotate 6 times in a counter clockwise direction gradually shrinking the circle until it returns to the navel.

Opening Up the Front and Back Energy Channels

The way to open the micro-cosmic energy channels is by sitting in meditation for a few minutes every day. Allow your energy to complete the loop by letting your mind flow along with it. At first it will feel like nothing is happening, but eventually the current will begin to feel warm in some places as it loops around. The key is simply to relax and try to bring your mind directly into the part of the loop being focused on (figure 6-3).

COMPLETING THE MICROCOSMIC ORBIT

The two channels form a single circuit that the energy loops around in circles. When this energy flows in a loop around the body through these two channels, the Chinese masters said the "small heavenly cycle or microcosmic orbit has been completed."

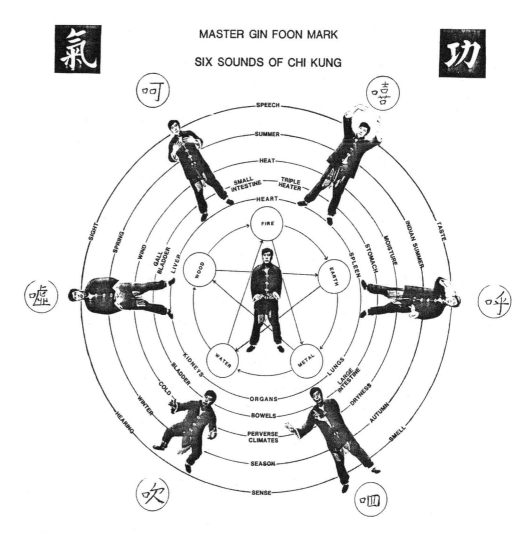

figure 6-3

CHAPTER 7
CONCLUSION

Qigong. The Chinese believe that true health depends on the well being of the internal organs and not on the external physique of the body. To this end they have developed sets of exercises called Qigong to improve and maintain the health of the internal organs. These exercises consist mainly of simple arm movements performed in conjunction with one's breathing. Qigong teaches students to become aware of their Qi (life force energy) and to circulate it through the acupuncture meridians of the body. The practice of Qigong can help reduce or normalize blood pressure, control diabetes, relieve fatigue, headaches, and much more. Results of such exercise systems are well documented in Chinese and Japanese hospitals.

Like Gongfu, there are also many styles of Qigong. Master Mark teaches Six Healing Sounds Qigong. In this style of Qigong each of the major internal organ systems has its own specific set of arm movements and breathing sounds (see figure 6-3). Using the sounds in conjunction with the arm movements helps to concentrate the beneficial effects on the desired organ. While all styles of Qigong are good, Six Healing Sounds Qigong is especially well suited for targeting specific problems as well as promoting overall good health.

If you have any questions concerning these Qigong exercises, or you are interested in learning directly from Master Mark, here is his contact information:

Master Gin Foon Mark
2259 Minnehaha Avenue
St. Paul, MN 55119
651-739-0778
www.masterginfoonmark.com

INDEX

BOOKS & VIDEOS FROM YMAA

YMAA Publication Center Books

YMAA Publication Center Videotapes

YMAA PUBLICATION CENTER 楊氏東方文化出版中心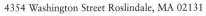

4354 Washington Street Roslindale, MA 02131

1-800-669-8892 • ymaa@aol.com • www.ymaa.com